You and Your Back

You and Your Back

by **Dr David Delvin** and edited by **Helene Grahame**
for the **Back Pain Association**

Pan Original
Pan Books London and Sydney

First published in Great Britain 1975
by the Back Pain Association Ltd
This revised edition published 1977 by Pan Books Ltd,
Cavaye Place, London SW10 9PG
© Back Pain Association Ltd 1975, 1977
ISBN 0 330 25065
Printed and bound in Great Britain by
Richard Clay (The Chaucer Press) Ltd, Bungay, Suffolk

Contents

Introduction

What does back trouble mean to you? Constant misery; an unforgettable, painful week; the odd twinge? Something that happens to somebody else? You may not, so far, have experienced it yourself, especially if you're young and fit. But did you realize how common it is?

Almost certainly, every year one in twenty-five people in Britain goes to the doctor about back pain. So even if you are lucky enough to escape, it's almost certain one of your family will run into some kind of back pain. At your workplace, four out of five of your colleagues will have back trouble at some stage in their careers.

It's not just men who run into these problems; women, too, get back disorders that incapacitate them for periods of time ranging from a day or two up to several weeks.

So there's no doubt that back pain is relevant *to you*. Even if you're never troubled by it yourself, it's odds on that one of your nearest and dearest will encounter it. And it's a certainty that many of your friends and relations will get it.

Well, that sounds a bit grim and gloomy, doesn't it? But let's get one thing clear right at the start:

Back pain isn't usually a sign of some really serious disease

It's a nuisance, it may be very unpleasant, it may be bad enough to keep you away from work or sport. But it's rarely a symptom of some dreadful disorder.

Now, that doesn't alter the fact that if you have *recurrent* back pain, or if you have a pain that interferes with work or other activities, then you *must* see your doctor. Back pain that goes on and on or keeps coming back, or back pain that is severe must not be ignored: in such circumstances, you've *got* to see your general practitioner – just in case something is wrong that needs medical attention.

But the great majority of backache cases are not due to anything serious: usually, the trouble is a temporary strain that will get better with rest or whatever else your doctor advises. He is the man to decide – don't try to 'out-diagnose' him with this book!

This book tells you about the important causes of back pain, ranging from the simple things like ligament and muscle strains that most people get at some time, to the less common forms of back disorder like so-called 'slipped discs'. It offers advice on how to cope with an acute attack of backache and how to come to terms with a back pain problem instead of living in perpetual fear and discomfort.

The book also tells you something about how back pain is treated, so that you'll know what's going to happen when you go to a doctor. So see him if you're worried, and especially if a bad attack of pain goes on for more than a day or two: – don't feel you have to grin and bear it! But don't rush off to your doctor just because you feel stiff and uncomfortable after an unusually hard day of gardening or spring cleaning. And just because you've had a bad attack of back pain don't think you're going to be crippled, or paralysed, or severely incapacitated – this just isn't true. If back pain is neglected, it can sometimes lead to quite serious troubles, but it's *not* a killer, and it usually responds to simple treatment arranged through your doctor.

Finally, this book tells you what is perhaps the most important thing of all – HOW TO AVOID BACK PAIN. *Most backache* is *preventable* and there's a very great deal in the old saying 'Prevention is better than cure'. While pain in the back can, in the great majority of cases, be cured you'll agree that it's an awful lot better to stop it happening in the first place.

And if you want to stop it happening, then read on ...

1 The normal back

One of the big problems that the average person runs into when he's trying to understand back trouble is that the back is a most complicated part of the body, with several different jobs to do.

The back is subjected to many strains – some are inevitable and others can be avoided or lessened if you take sensible precautions. Let's have a look at its structure and see how it's made up.

The spinal cord

First of all, let's be clear as to what we mean by the spinal cord. This isn't, as people often think, a part of the spine or backbone. As you can see from the drawing (figure 1), it's actually a continuation of the brain – a column of nerve tissue that runs down from the base of the skull to the level of the small of the back.

What does the spinal cord do? Well, basically, it's a relayer of messages. The roots of various nerves run out from it; these nerves supply the arms, the legs, the internal organs and, in fact, all the parts of the body.

When you decide to move (let's say) your leg, what happens is that your brain sends a message down the spinal cord and into the nerves which lead to the muscles in the leg. And when *they* get this signal, they move.

Messages travel in the opposite direction, too. If you tread on a drawing-pin, pain signals travel up the nerves from the foot and into the spinal cord, which carries them on up to

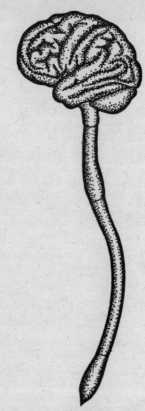

figure 1

the brain. Only when they arrive at the brain are you consciously aware of the pain.

So the spinal cord is basically the great communications channel of the body. If it's damaged – which takes a fairly severe injury – then you're in serious trouble. But, happily, hardly any of the various disorders causing back pain produce damage to the spinal cord.

The spinal column

Now, the spinal cord lies within a protective tunnel which runs through the spine, commonly called the spinal column or backbone.

You can see the spine in our next drawing (figure 2) – there it is, running down from just below the skull to end more or less at the top of the buttocks.

The first thing you'll notice is that it's made up of lots of little bones, each of which is called a vertebra. Every vertebra between the neck and the small of the back has a hole through it, so that there's a continuous tunnel for the spinal cord to pass through.

Now let's look at the general shape of the spine. You can see that it curves slightly forwards in the neck, slightly backwards in the chest, slightly forwards again in the small of the back, and backwards again in the lowest part of the spine. Doctors usually think of the spine as being split into five regions:

1 The cervical region This is the neck area, where the spine curves slightly forwards. It's also very *flexible* here, so that you can move your head backwards and forwards, or from side to side, or turn it.

In the cervical region, there are seven bones. As you can imagine, the joints between them are fairly complicated – they have to be, to allow for all these movements. In this area, degenerative changes are very common indeed in middle-aged and elderly people. Sometimes, though by no means always, these changes are associated with considerable pain, and sometimes the pain spreads to the shoulders, arms and hands.

2 The thoracic region This is the back of the chest area, where the normal spine curves *backwards*, without any twisting to

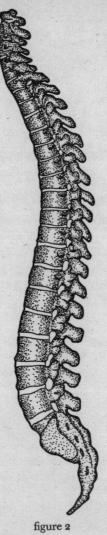

figure 2

left or right. Quite a few people do have a twist in the spine in this region, and this can cause pain and sometimes other problems as well.

Unlike the neck (cervical) region, this isn't a very flexible part of the spine. None of us, except contortionists, can achieve a great deal of movement between the bones here, and degenerative troubles in this part of the spine aren't very common, even among very old people.

There are twelve bones which go to make up the thoracic part of the spine, and they are rather larger and heavier than the bones in the neck region. The reason for this is that each vertebra in the thoracic region has attached to it not only a *rib* but also a number of *powerful muscles* which need something firm to pull against. When you do heavy work involving your arms, shoulders and upper trunk, the stresses on the bones in your thoracic spine are considerable. But, in fact, each of them does its job so effectively that back pain arising from injury to a thoracic vertebra, or from trouble arising in the joints between these bones, is rare.

3 The lumbar region This is the area of the 'small of the back'. Here, as we've said, the spine curves slightly forwards, and it's capable of bending backwards, forwards, and sideways. Stand upright and bow from the waist, then lean backwards as far as you can without strain and finally incline as far as you can first to one side and then the other. In all these manoeuvres, your *lumbar spine* is bending.

So the lumbar part of the spine, like the cervical spine up in the neck region, is very flexible indeed. And just like the cervical spine, the lumbar area is particularly prone to degenerative troubles in later life and even more to disc problems.

There are five bones which go to make up the lumbar spine, and they are all very big and very strongly built. Once

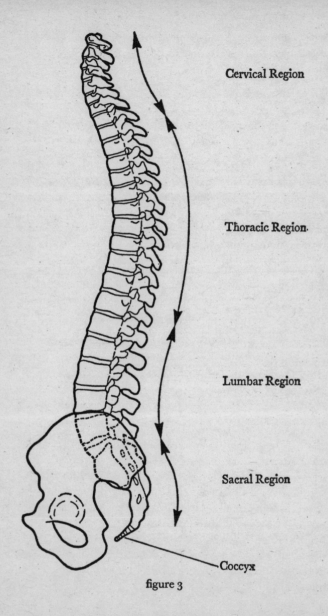

Cervical Region

Thoracic Region

Lumbar Region

Sacral Region

Coccyx

figure 3

again, many powerful muscles are attached to the spine in this region, and each vertebra has to be strong to withstand the stresses imposed on it.

4 The sacral region This is the area just above the buttocks where the spine curves backwards again. No significant movement is possible in this part of the spine, because the five little bones that make it up are fused together.

As you can see from the picture, (figure 3) this part of the spine is really part of the *pelvis* – the ring of bone that protects the delicate organs in the lower part of the body. In fact, one of the main functions of the sacral part of the spine is to provide protection from the rear for such structures as the womb, the bowel and the bladder.

5 The coccyx This is the very last and lowest part of the spine – the little bony bit that you can feel under the skin at the top of the cleft between the buttocks. It's formed from about four tiny little bones, on average.

In fact, the coccyx is the remnant of the tail found in primates like monkeys who use it to swing from tree to tree. It still has one function – to act as a fixing place for the attachment of certain muscle fibres. It can give trouble, however, and it's possible for backache to arise in this area after injury.

In particular, if you ever have the bad luck to fall heavily on to your bottom (the sort of thing that happens if somebody plays the foolish trick of whipping your chair away!), you may damage this little 'tail'. Severe pain that goes on for more than a few days after such a fall should always be reported to your doctor. An X-ray may be necessary, but often no fracture is seen, even though the pain may sometimes persist for months. But it usually goes away eventually; if it doesn't, steroid injections or manipulation may help.

The spinal nerves

We've said that the spinal cord is the great communications
channel of the body, and that it runs through a long tunnel
going down through the bones of the spine. We've also said
that the roots of these nerves flow in and out of it, taking
messages upwards and downwards.

But how do these spinal nerves get through the protective
bone to reach the spinal cord ? Well, they simply pass
through gaps between the bones (figure 4).

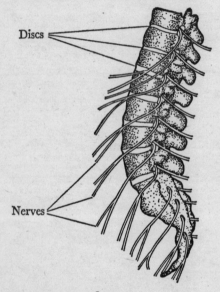

Discs

Nerves

figure 4

As you can imagine, there's not much room to spare in
these gaps, particularly when the person is bending over in
one direction or another, so it's not unknown for the nerves
to be *compressed*, especially when disc trouble is present (see
below). If there is pressure on a nerve, the person may

notice pain, numbness or tingling – which he will mentally register as occurring in the area of the body that the nerve supplies.

For instance, if a disc is pressing on a nerve which passes between two of the bones in the lumbar region (just as in the picture below), the result will often be pain felt *not* in the back, but down the leg(s), because the nerves in the lumbar region include those which carry pain impulses upwards from the leg – and this 'fools' the brain into thinking that the trouble is there!

The discs

But what actually are the famous discs? Well, they're shock-absorbers – fluid-filled cushions of cartilage (gristle) which lie between the bones of the spine, forming flexible pads that help to protect the whole structure against stresses.

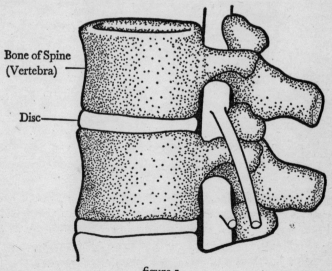

Bone of Spine (Vertebra)

Disc

figure 5

Each disc is made up of a fluid, jelly-like centre with a fibrous ring around it. This ring is weakest at the back and sides of the disc, and unfortunately there are times when it gives way, allowing the central jelly-like part to bulge out. If this bulge presses against one of the spinal nerves, (figure 6)

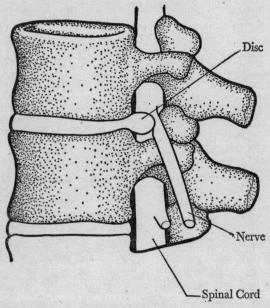

figure 6

the result is *pain*. We'll talk about disc trouble in Chapter 5 but you can see already that the term 'slipped disc' is an inaccurate one; a disc doesn't slip at all – it bulges.

Contrary to what many people believe, disc trouble isn't anywhere near the commonest cause of back pain. Some experts think it causes only about five-to-seven per cent of all cases of low backache.

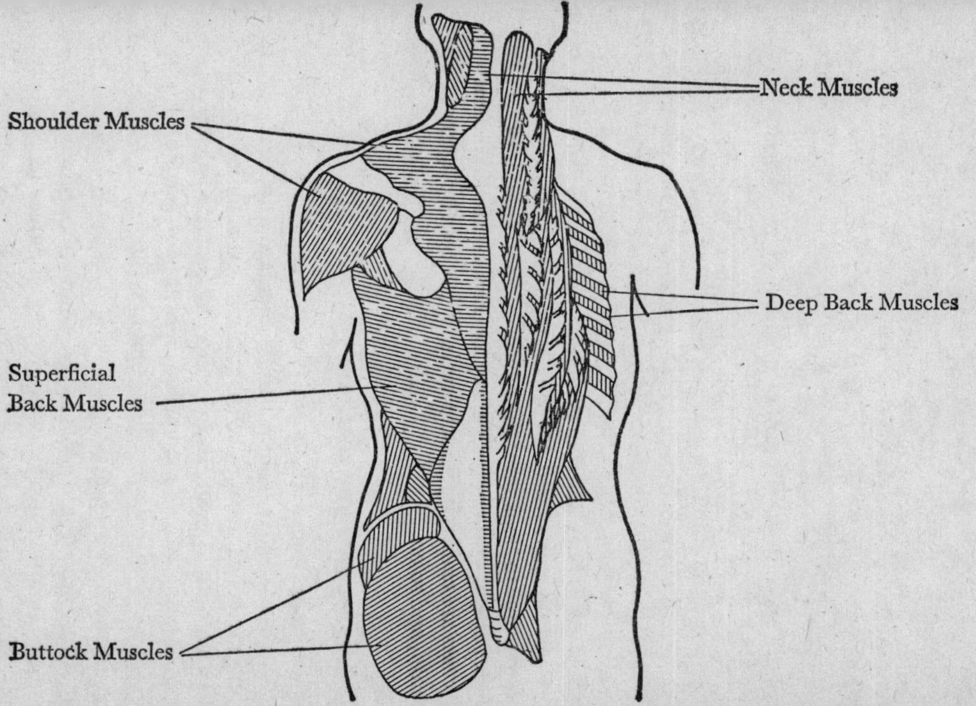

Neck Muscles

Deep Back Muscles

Shoulder Muscles

Superficial
Back Muscles

Buttock Muscles

figure 7

21

The muscles

A very large number of muscles, some big and powerful, some tiny and weak, are attached to the various bones of the spine.

When your body moves, these muscles contract, often throwing considerable strain on the spine.

However, most of the time, when something gives, it's the muscle fibres, or the fibres of ligaments or tendons (see below), not the spine.

This is a tremendously important point to appreciate, because what it means is this: *the majority of cases of backache are thought to be due to strains or 'fatigue' of these muscle fibres or to ligament strains and NOT to any serious disease*. It follows that most cases of backache will get better, provided the muscle strain is not aggravated. Of course, we must stress that it's not possible to 'look into' the back during an episode of back pain, so that no one can say for certain that X per cent of cases are caused by muscle strain, Y per cent by ligament strain, and so on.

The ligaments and tendons

The various bones of the back are bound together by bands of tough connective tissue called ligaments. No doubt you've seen ligaments (when slicing a chicken, for instance), as bands of thin, strong tissue – often with a rather silvery appearance – around the joints. There are also cords of strong connective tissue called tendons or sinews.

Ligaments and tendons often tear slightly, just like muscles, and this kind of ligamentous strain is also a very common cause of backache. In fact, though doctors differ widely on this point, some experts believe that ligament strains are more common causes of back pain. These strains, too, will get better, given a chance.

Finally, let's stress again:

Minor muscle and ligament strains are the cause of most cases of back pain. Serious causes are rare, and the so-called 'slipped disc' accounts for only a small percentage of cases.

2 When things go wrong . . .

In the last chapter we looked at the complex structure of the spine – a column of nearly three dozen irregularly shaped bones surrounded by muscles and ligaments, and containing within the column the spinal cord, the great communications channel that runs down from the brain.

It's a remarkable and highly efficient structure, yet things can go wrong with it. Why?

Well, one reason is the sheer complexity of the back: dozens of ligaments, bones, nerves and blood vessels fitted together in the most intricate way. It would be extremely difficult to design a piece of machinery like that, but if you did come up with something similar to it on a drawing board, it's a fair bet that you'd expect something to go wrong with it at times!

It is difficult to be at all certain of the other reasons why so many people are troubled by back disorders. All we can really say is that some experts believe that *it is actually the physical strains of modern life that make civilized humans, with their lesser degree of physical fitness, so liable to backache.*

This certainly seems a very likely explanation of why so many of us run into trouble with our backs – and *what that means is that back trouble is largely preventable.* All you have to do is to avoid some of the stresses that modern-day civilization puts on your spine, and maintain general muscular fitness – though perhaps that's easier said than done!

What sort of stresses are we talking about?

Obesity

Well, let's begin by looking at the stress caused by excess body weight. Obesity is to a very large extent a disease of modern civilization. In times gone by, it was really only the rich who could afford to be fat! In this country it's far and away the biggest nutritional problem of all – according to some estimates, almost half the adult population of Britain and the USA are carrying too much fat.

What's the effect on the spine of all this excess weight? Not good at all! If you imagine your spine as being something like a television mast swaying in the wind, and then think about what the effect would be of slinging a heavy weight on one side of the mast, about half-way down, (figure 8) well then you'll have some idea of what happens when a person's spine has to support a fat paunch in addition to its normal load! Incidentally, a similar situation occurs in women in the later stages of pregnancy, which is one reason why backache is common then.

We'll be dealing with what you can do if overweight is threatening your back, in Chapter 4.

Lifting

Ask the average person to lift a weight – say a tool box or a heavy shopping basket – from the floor and the odds are that he or she will do it in a way that is actually dangerous to the back. *There are right and wrong ways of lifting things*, and when so many people habitually choose the wrong way it's not surprising the result is very often a torn back muscle or torn ligament.

In fact, one could make a case for saying that Man (or Woman) really shouldn't do any lifting of heavy weights at all – and there's little doubt that if we did no lifting whatever there would be a lot less back pain about.

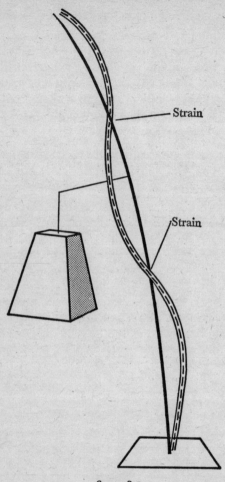

Strain

Strain

figure 8

But, of course, that just isn't practical – suitcases, toolboxes, shopping baskets and babies do have to be lifted. But when you lift them, the great thing is to use a relatively *safe* method that won't tear something and cause you days or weeks of agony. We'll look at these approved methods of lifting in Chapter 4.

Sitting

As with lifting, so with sitting: every time they use a chair, many, if not most, people sit in a way that may well lead to back trouble in the fullness of time. In Chapter 4 we'll look at correct ways of sitting.

But life isn't made any easier by the fact that *most of the chairs that we sit in are poorly designed from the point of view of back support.*

This applies to chairs at work, in the home, and on public transport – in fact, everywhere! For instance, you'd think that the airline seats used by pilots would be well designed. In fact, over half of pilots suffer from backache, and some of them have to use cushions and old socks stuffed with paper to make their seats comfortable! As for airline passenger seats, they just couldn't be worse, says one noted orthopaedic surgeon. If you've ever taken a long flight in an aircraft, you'll probably agree with him. But, really, seats elsewhere are just as bad – so in Chapter 4 we'll be looking at the sort of chair you ought to select in order to keep you from getting backache.

Driving

Sitting in a car or lorry, particularly as the driver, is by and large not good for the back – but unfortunately it's one of those activities that civilized man finds it hard to do without!

Not only are car seats, like other seats, poorly designed for support of the back, but the posture which many people take up when they're at the wheel is very bad for their spines. That's one reason why taxi and bus drivers and commercial travellers get a lot of back trouble. When we come to Chapter 4 we'll also look at the best ways of minimizing back strain if you have to do a lot of travelling by car.

Bending and stretching

Watch a class of children being put through 'physical jerks'. Very often you'll see them being told to do something that many experts think is not good at all for the back – touching the toes without bending the knees.

But it's not just in PE classes that human beings carry out this kind of movement. In picking up things off the floor at work, in cleaning the house and making beds, in doing the garden – time and again people bend forwards without flexing the knees, and so put a severe strain on the back. No wonder that sometimes something 'goes'.

In the next chapter, we'll be looking at bending and stretching movements that could be dangerous to your back – and discussing ways in which you can avoid these unnecessary stressful movements.

Poor posture

Most people in this country don't pay enough attention to posture, which is why so many of us slop about round-shouldered and slouching. We've already talked about posture in the sitting position, but good posture when standing is important, too.

If children aren't taught correct posture, they very often develop slight curvatures of the spine or tilting of the pelvis – and these malpositions can easily lead to severe back trouble later on. Much of the success of Yoga practitioners in dealing with backache has been due to their ability to show people that they are standing badly, and to get them to hold themselves correctly. We'll try to do the same for you in the next chapter.

Beds

Once upon a time, primitive man slept on dry bracken, or on a pile of animal skins thrown on the floor of a cave. Nowadays, most of us sleep on beds that are far more comfortable – but probably far more dangerous for our backs!

In fact, most modern beds are *far too soft*. They give too much and don't support the spine properly. This is why, very often, when a man has to take to his bed because of back pain, the doctor will advise him to have a board put under his mattress.

Exercise

Although one shouldn't strain the spine by stressful movements, there's no doubt that inactivity, too, is bad for the back. Perhaps this is another reason why people who spend much of their working lives behind a driving wheel get backache.

Everybody, except for invalids, really needs a certain amount of physical exertion each day to keep the muscles and ligaments in a healthy state, and the man or woman who gets insufficient exercise is laying up a store of trouble as far as health is concerned. Exercise is good, not only for the back muscles and ligaments, but also for the heart, the circulation, the lungs and the body generally. In Chapter 4 we'll tell you a little about the sort of exercises you can take that will help to keep you, and your back, in tip-top condition.

Accidents and falls

Of course, very often things begin to go wrong in somebody's back as a result of an accident or a fall. (Curiously enough, the backache may not start at the time of the accident, but come on a few hours, a few days, or even sometimes a week or two later.)

It's easy to say that you should avoid accidents if you want to avoid backache. Easier said than done! But it's quite true that if we all took a bit more care and thought a bit more about safety precautions (particularly at work) then there would be fewer accidents and fewer back injuries.

For instance, if the safety regulations at your workplace say that you shouldn't climb something without a safety harness, or shouldn't lift something without help, then follow them! If there are heavy loads stacked at work or on a lorry which you drive, always make sure that they're properly secured. And don't stand around in places where loads or other falling objects could slip and come down on you – every year people suffer fractures of the spine as a result of accidents of this sort. Unfortunately, some of them end up with not just back pain, but paralysis for life.

Accidents on the road are also a major cause of back injuries, so we need hardly say how just a little bit more care by everybody on the road could reduce our national toll of back pain. In particular, you can minimize your chances of back injury from a road accident by wearing your seatbelt, by having a properly designed car seat, and by using a good head restraint (not the inadequate and dangerous type which so many people have in their cars). Seats and head restraints are discussed in Chapter 4.

Accidents and falls also cause a lot of back injuries among sportsmen and sportswomen. This kind of thing is certainly hard to avoid, since it's very easy for a sudden jolt to give you a back strain. But a person who's physically fit and in good training stands less chance of sustaining a painful muscle or ligament injury than someone who just goes in for sport without any adequate preparation. Many of the 'bad backs' which turn up in doctors' surgeries are caused by accidents or falls which have happened to people who haven't done any proper training for their sport. The opening of the cricket season is a prime time for this sort of thing!

Finally, there's one group of people who should be *specially* careful about avoiding falls and accidents and that's the elderly. Older people are particularly liable to strain their backs (and other parts of their bodies) if they fall. They should take extra care in wet or icy weather to avoid taking a tumble.

Overdoing it

Perhaps the most important message to remember where backache is concerned is: *don't overdo things.* The back (as many of us know to our cost) is a sensitive part of the body, and dislikes being overexerted. The common mistakes that people make are: overdoing the housework (if your back is beginning to hurt, then leave the rest of the polishing till next day); overdoing the gardening (the rest of the weeds will wait until tomorrow) and lifting too much. In any activity, once you get the 'danger signal' of pain or discomfort in the back, then it's time to stop!

Triggering off old strains

Unfortunately, if you've had back trouble in the past you're quite likely to trigger off another attack in the future. So, if you've got a history of back trouble, then you must take special care (more than the average person) to avoid the kinds of strain we've been talking about. Unfortunately, though, it's true that the sufferer from recurrent back pain can sometimes trigger off a repeat attack by the most trivial of movements – turning over in bed, stretching to open a car door, or indeed even sneezing!

3 How to cope with an acute attack

What on earth do you do when back pain strikes? What's the best course of action in those first few hours after it hits you? This is an important topic: few people know what the best 'first aid' for back pain is. So, when it hits them they may try to soldier on (and so make things worse) or try some remedy that really won't be the least help. In fact, sensible measures, taken at the very outset of an attack, will help keep pain and disability to a minimum, or even abort the attack altogether.

Immediate action

If you get a severe back pain, then you must stop all physical activity right away. Your back is giving you urgent warning signals that something is wrong, and it's quite crazy to disregard the message.

So, if intense pain hits you while you're working or doing the housework, then *stop*. If you're at your workplace, then go home – preferably getting a lift in a car rather than fighting your way there by public transport. If your employer is sensible, he probably won't mind – after all, it's better for both of you if you take a single day off at the onset of an attack than if you have to take four weeks off because you've ignored the warning signals.

Pain-killers

The next thing to do is to take a pain-killer. Which one? The choice isn't difficult – it's simply a question of deciding between an aspirin-containing pain-killer and a paracetamol-containing one. The two kinds are of roughly equal strength in relieving pain.

Aspirin is available as 'ordinary' aspirin tablets, as soluble aspirin, and under various proprietary names. Most doctors do not believe that there is any great difference between the various types of preparation, and ordinary aspirin bought from your chemist is certainly cheap and effective. The usual dose is two tablets, three or four times a day, preferably after meals – but you shouldn't continue this dosage of aspirin or any other pain-killer for more than a few days without seeking medical advice.

Side-effects

Most people can take aspirin with perfect safety. But sometimes it may cause tummy pain or even (rarely) internal bleeding. So if you get any tummy discomfort when you use aspirin (or if you've had a gastric or duodenal ulcer) *don't* use aspirin without discussing things with your doctor – take a paracetamol-containing preparation instead.

(*Note:* you can check whether a proprietary preparation contains aspirin by seeing if the words 'acetysalicylic acid' or a similar abbreviation appear on the side of the pack. Sometimes manufacturers do not make it clear that the main pain-killing ingredient of their product is in fact aspirin!)

Paracetamol is also a good pain-killer. Again, the dose is two tablets three or four times a day. This drug does not produce tummy irritation but, like aspirin, it can be dangerous if an overdose (say 10 to 20 tablets for an adult) is taken. So don't leave either kind of tablet lying around the house.

Going to bed

In a severe attack of back pain, you should go to bed and keep warm. Nothing is sillier than sitting around the house watching TV and hoping the pain will go away. It probably won't.

So go to bed and stay there, except when you have to get up to go to the toilet. In fact, in a bad attack, it may be easier for you to crawl along the floor to the loo on all fours rather than to try to walk there.

We'll be saying more about beds later in this book. But if your mattress is the least bit soft, then that could be a bad thing for your back. If in doubt, ask somebody to shove a firm board underneath it (please don't try and do this yourself – you're meant to be resting!). Some people find that in an acute attack the best way to get relief is to have the bedclothes 'made up' on the floor, because this is the only thing that's firm enough.

Making yourself warm and comfortable

Anyone in an acute attack of backache is entitled to be cosseted a bit! This means that the rest of the family must be prepared to bring you meals and cups of tea in bed. They should also be willing to get you hot water bottles – these may be of considerable value in helping to relieve the pain during those first few unpleasant hours.

Also, get one of the family to experiment with placing pillows (or, better, old-fashioned bolsters) alongside you. Usually it's best to lie flat on your back, but if you're reasonably comfortable on your side, then a pillow or bolster in the small of the back may help.

Above all, do be careful when turning over and reaching for things from bedside tables. Make all movements slowly – a sudden twist can easily make the back strain much worse, and it's far better to ask somebody to help and support you *before* you move.

Seeking skilled help

Now, how soon should you call the doctor? This is a difficult one to answer, but, in general, there is nothing urgent or immediate that a doctor can do in the first few hours of an attack. So there's no point in doing what I'm afraid one or two people with back pain do – summon their GP even if it's the middle of the night, insisting that he come at once. As a rule, all the poor doctor can do is offer the same sort of advice that we've given here, and prescribe a pain-killer.

But you certainly should let your doctor know after twelve hours or so if you've got a really bad attack of back pain. If you talk to him on the phone he'll advise you about how soon you should be seen and whether it will be safe for you to come down to the surgery, or if he should come and see you first.

The subject of help from an osteopath or chiropractor is discussed later in the book, but if you're going to contact an osteopath in these early stages of the attack, mention this to your doctor. Remember that osteopaths are very busy nowadays and that many of them are booked up for a week or more, so that you may have to wait a while for an appointment.

Continuing care

Once the doctor has seen you, do follow his advice about
how long you should stay in bed. Quite frequently, a GP
will advise his patient to stay lying down for at least a week –
and I'm afraid that all too often his advice is disregarded!
However important you feel it is to get back to your work
(or housework), please do remain in that nice, warm bed
till the doctor says that it's safe to start moving around
again.

Incidentally, you don't have to remain perfectly still in
bed – indeed, if you do so over a period of days you might
risk getting a clot in your leg veins. To avoid this, it's best
to make a point of moving your legs around while you're
confined to bed. Three half-hour periods of gentle leg
exercise each day should be sufficient.

4 How to prevent back pain

(*Note:* While this chapter is about preventive measures for people who've never had back pain, the tips in it should also be used by those who are already back pain sufferers.)

We've said that civilized man largely brings back pain on himself by subjecting his back to unnecessary stresses, and by allowing his muscles to get flabby through lack of exercise.

But how can *you* avoid these stresses? Let's take them one by one ...

Don't get overweight

... and if you already *are* overweight, then start dieting now! The table below gives you an idea of what weight you should be for your height. If you're more than, say, 4·5 kg (10 lb) above the recommended weight, then we suggest that you contact your GP and ask him for a diet sheet. Please don't try to pressurize him into giving you slimming pills, which are of limited value and – in some cases – dangerous. If you really cut your food intake sufficiently and take active exercise, as advised by your doctor, you're bound to lose weight. If you have difficulty, your GP can refer you to the local hospital dietician. Alternatively, you could contact Weight Watchers (look them up in the phone book). Remember that weight comes *only* from the food you eat and the liquid – especially alcohol – that you drink. (See our ideal weights and heights chart below.)

Ideal weights and heights: women
(in indoor clothes, without shoes)

Height	Large build	Medium build	Small build
147 cm (4 ft 10 in)	51·0 kg (8 st)	47·5 kg (7 st 7 lb)	44·5 kg (7 st)
152 cm (5 ft)	53·5 kg (8 st 6 lb)	51·0 kg (8 st)	47·5 kg (7 st 7 lb)
157 cm (5 ft 2 in)	56·5 kg (8 st 13 lb)	53·5 kg (8 st 6 lb)	50·5 kg (7 st 13 lb)
163 cm (5 ft 4 in)	59·0 kg (9 st 4 lb)	56·0 kg (8 st 12 lb)	53·0 kg (8 st 5 lb)
168 cm (5 ft 6 in)	61·5 kg (9 st 10 lb)	58·0 kg (9 st 2 lb)	54·5 kg (8 st 8 lb)
173 cm (5 ft 8 in)	65·0 kg (10 st 3 lb)	61·0 kg (9 st 9 lb)	56·5 kg (8 st 13 lb)
178 cm (5 ft 10 in)	68·0 kg (10 st 10 lb)	64·5 kg (10 st 2 lb)	60·5 kg (9 st 7 lb)
183 cm (6 ft)	71·0 kg (11 st 3 lb)	67·5 kg (10 st 9 lb)	63·5 kg (10 st)

Ideal weights and heights: men
(in indoor clothes, without shoes)

Height	Large build	Medium build	Small build
163 cm (5 ft 4 in)	63·5 kg (10 st)	60·0 kg (9 st 6 lb)	57·5 kg (9 st 1 lb)
168 cm (5 ft 6 in)	67·5 kg (10 st 9 lb)	64·0 kg (10 st 1 lb)	61·0 kg (9 st 9 lb)
173 cm (5 ft 8 in)	73·5 kg (11 st 8 lb)	70·0 kg (11 st)	66·0 kg (10 st 5 lb)
178 cm (5 ft 10 in)	78·0 kg (12 st 4 lb)	74·0 kg (11 st ~9 lb)	69·5 kg (10 st 13 lb)
183 cm (6 ft)	83·5 kg (13 st 2 lb)	78·0 kg (12 st 4 lb)	73·0 kg (11 st 7 lb)
188 cm (6 ft 2 in)	89·0 kg (14 st)	83·0 kg (13 st 1 lb)	77·0 kg (12 st 2 lb)
193 cm (6 ft 4 in)	93·0 kg (14 st 9 lb)	87·5 kg (13 st 11 lb)	80·5 kg (12 st 9 lb)

Lifting

Try to avoid lifting heavy weights – i.e. anything over about
10 kg (20–25 lb). If you *have* to shift something heavier than
this, try to use some alternative technique instead of lifting.

For instance, if you have to move a wardrobe or a chest of
drawers (and you should get help for such a task), it's quite
easy to manipulate it by slipping your foot under it; all you
do is to leave your heel on the ground and raise the front
part of your foot underneath the piece of furniture
(figure 9). Similarly, many loads can be shifted by just
sliding them along, or getting a trolley underneath, instead
of lifting them (figure 10).

If you *must* lift something, try to use a technique that doesn't involve the lumbar spine at all. For instance, if an object is carried on the front of the hip bone (figure 11) there is very little stress on the lumbar spine. Similarly a

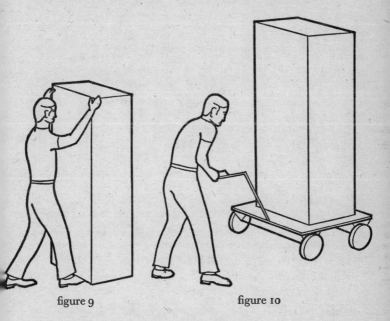

figure 9   figure 10

table can be lifted by simply putting the knee under it and bringing the thigh upwards (figure 12).

But of course there are times when most of us are obliged to lift something fairly heavy, say, a box full of shopping, with our arms. If you can't break the load up in some way and carry it in two or three trips instead of one, then do please protect your back by using the correct lifting techniques shown in the drawings. Most people automatically choose the techniques shown in the 'wrong' drawings – and lifting things this way is very, very bad for the back.

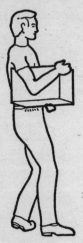

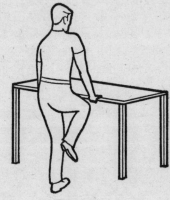

figure 11   figure 12

Why is this? Well, let's look at the drawings carefully
(figure 13). The basic difference between the 'right' ones
and the 'wrong' ones is that in the 'right' ones *the lifter is
lifting with a straight back*. In the 'wrong' illustrations, the
back is bent – and this puts great strain on the muscles,
tendons and ligaments around the spine, as well as exposing
the lifter to the risk of disc trouble.

Taking the pictures one by one, look at the 'wrong'
illustration of a man picking up a weight from the ground.
With his legs practically straight, he bends his spine
forwards and lifts the box with outstretched arms. Immense
tension is thereby placed on his lumbar spine, and it
wouldn't be surprising if, a moment later, he was clutching
his back in agony!

Now look at the chap who's lifting the right way. He has
bent his knees in order really to get down to the level of the
box. His back is straight, so that there is comparatively
little strain on it and (very important this) he's got his arms
bent so that the load is in close to his body.

It's a fact not generally known that *your arms are much stronger if they're close to your body*. Interestingly enough, this is one of the basic principles of judo – in which a man will rarely try to lift his opponent off the ground unless he has first pulled him in close against him. This same principle should be used when lifting *any* weight!

Now to the pictures of the lady lifting the baby from the cot (figure 14). The first thing to point out is that this cot is

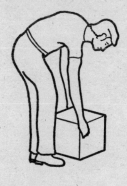   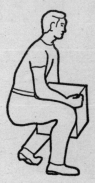

Wrong   Right

figure 13

far, far too low anyway! To keep having to pick a youngster up from this level is positively inviting back strain.

But obviously you can't avoid picking up kiddies from this height sometimes. So, if you have to do it, then don't bend at the waist like the lady in the 'wrong' picture. Instead, bend your knees until your elbows are right down at the level of the baby – then lift by simply straightening the legs. In lifting *always try to let the legs do the work* – they're much more capable of coping with it than the back is.

(*Note :* if the cot has a side that lowers, always let it down first.)

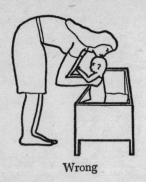
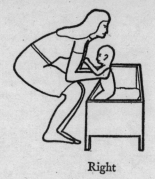

| Wrong | Right |

figure 14

Sitting

Here are two more 'right' and 'wrong' drawings
(figure 15). Once again, the slouching posture that so many
people adopt when in a chair is very bad for the spine.

You see, if your spine is bent over like this, it puts excessive
strain on all the muscles and ligaments that lie behind it –
and sooner or later they are going to start complaining!

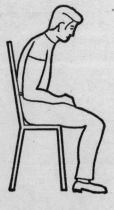
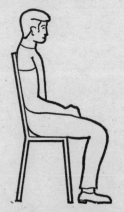

| Wrong | Right |

figure 15

Train your children, too, to sit up properly like the figure in the 'right' diagram – but note that this doesn't mean sitting to attention like a child in a Victorian classroom!

Seat design

The tendency that most people have to slump in their chairs isn't helped by the fact that most chairs are not well designed to accommodate the human form.

So what should you look for when choosing a chair? Here we're up against a difficulty because, although a massive amount of work is now being carried out on the design of seating, much research still remains to be done, and experts tend to disagree about some aspects of chair design.

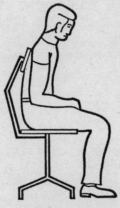

figure 16

However, virtually all authorities are agreed that most chairs on sale today do not give adequate support to the spine and especially to the lower portion of it. Many are far, far too soft, and others are so designed that the back of the chair scarcely comes into contact with the spine at all (figure 16).

Some experts believe that Man's spine was never really designed for sitting, anyway, but that if we have to sit, then we should always use chairs whose backs have an 'S-curve' to fit into the small of the back (figure 17).

In practice, you'll find it's difficult to buy a chair that does this, particularly as the bends of the 'S' may be at different levels in different people. But you can, if you wish, buy a lumbar support cushion that fits neatly into the curve of the lower spine and is certainly very comfortable to use.

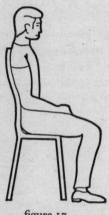
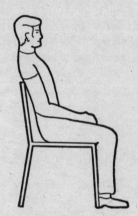

figure 17   figure 18

Other authorities disagree about the 'S-curve' theory but, in general, they do agree that the back of the chair should be in firm contact with the sitter's backbone. It is certainly courting trouble to sit for year after year in a chair that leaves your spine 15 cm (6 in) away from the back of the seat – as many typists do, for instance.

Now one thing that tends to keep your back too far from the chair back is the *depth of the seat*. In most modern chairs the seat is about 50 cm (19½ in), i.e. from front to back. But the average person's thigh is much shorter than this. The distance from the back of the knee to the back of the sitting part of the buttock is roughly 43 cm (17 in) in men and 38 cm (15 in) in women – which means, as you can see from the diagram, that most people find difficulty in getting far back enough to have the base of the spine resting against the bottom of the chair back (figure 18).

It's also important to remember that *a chair must be correctly adjusted in height for the job it's got to do*. All too often, people are given office or workbench chairs or stools that just aren't at the best height for them to do their work in comfort. If you sit at a desk or workbench, make sure the height of your chair is right in relation to the working surface. There's no hard and fast rule that we can make about the height of chairs – all we can say is that if you have to sit in an awkward position to do your work, or if you start feeling strain in your back when you've been sitting for any length of time, then it's essential to make sure that the height of your chair is right for *you*. If it's not, then ask for another one.

When you're driving

If you've got back trouble, it's usually best to avoid driving if you possibly can. Man's backbone wasn't meant to cope with the position we have to take up behind the wheel of a car – especially if the pedals are offset from the line of the seat.

However, if you have to drive, whether you've got back trouble or not, do try to sit in an upright posture that puts the least possible strain on the spine. Don't sit like the man in the 'wrong' picture here (figure 19), hunched forward over the wheel with knees sharply bent, because doing this widens the gap between the little bones of the spine and increases the tension on the various muscles and ligaments that keep these bones in correct alignment.

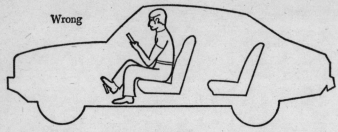

Wrong

figure 19

So, do try to sit like the man in the 'right' picture (figure 20), with back supported upright and straight, and legs extended.

Everything we've said about ordinary seats applies also to car seats. If you're buying a car, do think about the car seat. Try to choose a seat that gives firm support to your back while your hands are on the wheel – not one with a soft, cushiony seat that you sink into. If the lower part of the seat-back doesn't seem to be supporting the small of your back adequately, then get yourself a lumbar support cushion (figure 21).

Furthermore, you should bear in mind that in most cars the back rest of the seat doesn't come far enough up the spine – as a rule, it ends somewhere between the shoulder-blades, which is far too low.

The best place for the top of a car seat is *right behind the top*

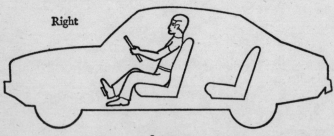

Right

figure 20

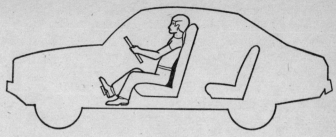

figure 21

of your head as shown in the drawing (figure 22). If this isn't the case with your car, then we suggest that you get a neck support fitted to the top of the seat. But please don't get the

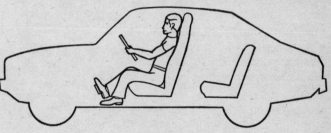

figure 22

sort of neck support that only comes up to the base of your skull (figure 23). These are dangerous and may damage your upper spine if your car is struck from behind or in front.

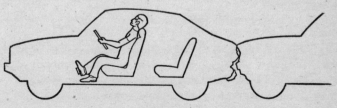

figure 23

The seat is often the last thing that most people think of when they buy a car. Bearing in mind that so much back pain is caused by driving, we think that the seat should be one of the first things that you look at.

Bending and stretching

A good deal of back pain may also be provoked by subjecting the back to stressful and unnecessary movements – particularly bending and stretching. This is so both in industry and in the home. A workman may find that the loads he has to lift are usually placed near the floor, or above, where he has to stretch for them. The housewife may have units in her kitchen arranged so that she has either to bend right down or to stretch on tiptoe perhaps forty or fifty times a day. Similarly, a secretary may have the filing cabinet drawer that she uses most frequently so near the floor that she too is bending dozens of times each day.

This is quite crazy – and it could all be prevented with a little planning. Just try to get the work surface (or cupboard or filing cabinet) that you use most at a height from the ground you find comfortable. Somewhere about 76 cm to 107 cm (2 ft 6 in to 3 ft 6 in) is usually best for most tasks, depending on whether they are undertaken in a sitting or standing position – and, of course, depending on the height of the person involved.

For this is the really crucial thing to grasp – that a surface which is just right for somebody of a different height probably *isn't* going to be comfortable for you. Let's take a very simple demonstration of this: most home washbasins are installed by builders at what they feel to be an 'average' height; in practice, what this means is that the basin is fitted low enough for a child to be able to reach it.

But what happens when a 1·9 metre (6 ft 4 in) man wants to shave at the washbasin? Any tall man with backache will tell you! Bending over a washbasin that is far too low can put a severe strain on the lumbar spine. Yet countless men must bend over bathroom basins that are too low for them, every morning of their lives: the only surprising thing is that many of them take ten to twenty years to develop that agonizing lumbar backache.

And as far as kitchen worktops are concerned, remember that the British Standard of 91 cm (3 ft) off the ground is not ideal for everybody. In a kitchen, worktops are most convenient at about 7·50 cm (3 in) below the rim of the sink, which, for most women, means about 94 cm to 107 cm (3 ft 1 in to 3 ft 6 in) above the floor, depending on your height. As to cupboards, a recent survey for *Which?* magazine by the Institute for Consumer Ergonomics suggested that, unless a housewife is unusually tall, her cupboards shouldn't start at more than 33 cm (13 in) above the worktops – and that no kitchen shelves should be more than 164 cm (5 ft 4½ in) off the ground.

It may not be necessary to shift all the furniture and fittings around to achieve economy of movement. For instance, if a housewife has units or shelves that are too high for her to stretch up to with ease, and if she can't afford to have them moved, then it's best if she works out what kitchen items (cornflakes, tins or whatever) she needs most frequently. These objects should be placed on more accessible shelves, say 91 cm (3 ft) off the ground. Things that she won't need very often (perhaps spices, herbs or sauces) can be relegated to the awkwardly placed units – and when she does need to get these things out, then, of course, she should use a properly constructed footstool (figure 24), not one of your old soap boxes, please!

One particular problem may be bed-making – a lot of modern divan beds are far too low off the floor: the answer

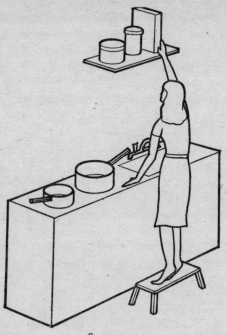

figure 24

here for the person with a tendency to backache is to buy a Continental duvet, get a new bed, or to kneel while making the bed if this is possible.

Sensible planning like this can prevent a lot of backache. But if you do have to lift things from very low surfaces, please use the techniques we've described, rather than just bending over and hauling them up.

Posture generally

In this country little emphasis is placed on posture, especially in childhood, though it's encouraging that quite a lot of women now go to posture classes, and that many women and men have taken up Yoga.

We can't deal with the whole subject of posture in a short book like this, but as you can see from the 'right' and 'wrong' pictures, the important thing, whether you're standing, walking, kneeling or whatever, is not to slouch around with hunched shoulders and tummy stuck out.

You don't have to hold yourself in a sort of 'sergeant-major' pose either, with chest thrust out and shoulders

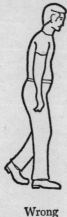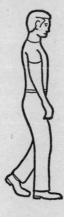

Wrong   Right

figure 25

exaggeratedly far back. All you have to do when you're standing is to keep your shoulders reasonably far back, your chest reasonably firmly pushed forwards, and your tummy reasonably pulled in. Above all, *try to keep your back upright* rather than bent forwards. Some authorities believe that the lower part of the back should be deliberately pushed forwards in an accentuation of the normal S-curve, but not all experts agree with this.

It is just as important to think about good posture if you have to do a job on the floor or at a very low level. When you are working below knee level – as when laying a carpet or cleaning the bath – it is sensible to do it from a kneeling

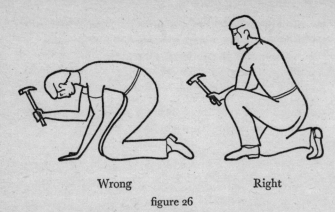

Wrong   Right

figure 26

position. But there is even a right way and a wrong way to kneel (figure 26). The right way is to go down on one knee and try to keep your back as straight as you can.

Beds

Here, our advice is brief and simple. If you want to avoid back pain, *choose a mattress that is really firm* – not one that you sink into. There are, in fact, very few mattresses on the market that really are firm enough to support the back properly.

It is best to buy your bed or mattress from a reputable manufacturer. Remember that you spend a third of your life in bed, and that a cheap mattress may well lose what firmness it has quite quickly. You should also be very wary about buying a second-hand bed or mattress: if it's had a few years of use, there is every chance that the support it gives will be seriously impaired. If you have to buy second-hand, always feel carefully all over the mattress with the flat of your hand, checking especially carefully the areas where the previous occupant or occupants have been lying night after night. If you feel any sensation of 'giving' or weakness, in these areas, don't buy! And don't forget

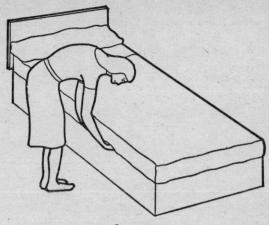

figure 27

that a high bed, fitted bottom sheet and Continental duvet
will make bed-making easier.

Exercise

Lack of exercise is one of the curses of Western civilization.
Not only is exercise good for your general health – unless,
of course, you're an invalid – but it's good for your back
muscles and ligaments, too.

Obviously, it's crazy to start taking violent exercise without
any preparation at all, particularly if you're no longer in the
first flush of youth. But gradually increasing exercise is good
for almost everybody – and to do you most good this
exercise should be daily, and not just once a week or so.

Useful exercises that can be done by almost anybody
include:

walking
swimming (especially good)
yoga

53

dancing
jogging (but check with your GP first if you're over forty)

For those who are fitter, good ways of getting exercise
include:

tennis
badminton
squash
judo
cycling (but watch the hills if you're over forty)
riding

One question that's often asked: is golf good exercise? The
answer is perhaps, because it gets you out and makes you
walk several miles in every round. Playing golf the
American-executive way, with buggies to take you round
the course, is absolutely pointless. On the other hand, golf
doesn't give active enough exercise to speed up the pulse
and respiration rate – something that really good exercise
should do.

Another point against golf is that carrying a heavy bag,
which is obligatory on all courses in winter unless you have
a caddy, isn't good for the back. If you have established
back trouble, you should ask your doctor's advice before
playing a lot of golf and, indeed, before going in for any of
the sports mentioned above. By reducing the number of
clubs to, say, six in all, and using a very light bag, you can
still have good sport and exercise – provided your doctor is
happy for you to play.

5 What kinds of back trouble are there?

Let's begin by saying that this chapter isn't intended to be a do-it-yourself guide to diagnosis! Please don't use it to try and 'out-diagnose' your doctor: after all, learning how to spot the likeliest cause of a pain in the back is a very skilled business that takes years of study – and it's still far from an exact science. Although most backache is 'mechanical' in origin, it can occasionally be a sign of serious disease requiring treatment. Your doctor is the best person to decide what's wrong with you if you have backache, so be guided by him.

But please do also bear in mind the fact that if your GP *can't* give you a precise diagnosis of what's wrong with your back, this doesn't mean that he's incompetent! Far too many people want their doctor to use important-sounding terms like 'lumbago' or 'sciatica', simply because they feel relieved to have a diagnosis made; but as we'll discover in a moment, lumbago and sciatica aren't disorders (as so many of us think) – they're just words that describe particular kinds of pain. To say that a back pain is 'due to lumbago' is quite meaningless.

The fact is that in many (if not most) cases of backache, it is difficult for a doctor to make an exact, scientific diagnosis of the cause of the trouble. All he can do is offer a reasonably well-informed opinion as to whether the pain might be due to one of various causes.

Why is this? It's because the back is not only one of the

most complicated areas of the body, but also *one of the most inaccessible to direct vision*. All sorts of organs can nowadays be inspected by surgeons, using slim, telescope-like instruments (for instance, the stomach, the bladder, the rectum, the abdominal cavity, and even the insides of large joints). But there is no way that a doctor can look into your *back* and tell you precisely what is going on there – except on the (comparatively rare) occasions when the back is opened up during a surgical operation.

Nor are X-rays as much help in diagnosis as most people imagine. By and large, X-rays show only bones, and are of little or no use in demonstrating what is going on in the *soft* tissues of the back, such as the muscles, ligaments and tendons.

So the human back remains something of an enigma. And when something goes wrong with it, all you can reasonably expect of your doctor is fairly general guidance – at least in the early stages. He'll tell you whether he thinks the trouble is serious or not, and whether he thinks it's likely to be long lasting. If he *can* pinpoint a precise diagnosis, he will do so – and if you don't understand what he means, ask him.

Most people are pretty bewildered by the terms used in describing various kinds of back trouble and particularly by the more inaccurate and misleading terms like 'lumbago', 'fibrositis', 'rheumatism' and 'slipped disc'. So what we'll do here is to try and put you in the picture about the various common types of back trouble. Then, if you or one of your family has one of these conditions, you'll have a better idea of what it's all about.

The regions of the spine

You may remember from Chapter 1 that the spine is divided into various regions: Cervical (neck), Thoracic (chest), Lumbar (small of back), Sacral and Coccygeal (the two lowest parts).

In the same chapter, we discussed the fact that, throughout life, the spine is subjected to a great deal of movement in just two of these regions – the neck, and the small of the back. In the other regions, there's relatively little movement in any direction.

Now the interesting thing is that it is *in just these two regions that back pain is commonest.* Though aches and pains do occur in the less flexible regions of the spine they're not so frequent.

So, although it's impossible to prove, many authorities do think that pain is common in these two areas (the neck and the lumbar region) *because of the amount of bending and twisting and turning under load they have to undergo – year in, year out.*

This tends to reinforce the main message of this book: if you can cut down on stressful movements of the spine, you'll probably also reduce your chances of backache.

Common disorders

Now . . . let's look at the common disorders that affect the back. Don't worry if you've never heard of some of them – they are still, in most cases, a good deal commoner than the famous so-called 'slipped disc' of which everyone's heard!

Muscle strain

As we said earlier in this booklet there are a very large number of muscles in the back, some big and powerful, some small and weak. These muscles are subjected to tremendous strains, particularly when we lift heavy weights or make sudden and awkward movements.

In such circumstances it's very easy indeed for a few fibres of muscle to tear – or perhaps to be ripped off the bone they are attached to. In such cases, the tear may involve the tendon attached to the muscle: in this case the symptoms and effects are similar to those of torn ligaments (see below).

So that's what a 'muscle strain' means.

It's often very painful but it's NOT serious.

In general, the pain comes on at the moment when the tear occurs but this isn't an invariable rule and it's quite common for a man who tears a few muscle fibres, say while gardening, not to notice any pain for a day or so.

Muscle strains are widely believed, together with ligament and tendon strains, to be the commonest cause of backache. It's probable that most are provoked by lifting – either lifting weights that are too heavy, or lifting with a poor technique (see Chapter 4).

The next chapter discusses treatment of back pain in general, but as a rule doctors encourage patients with muscle strains to keep mobile, rather than to take to their beds, though violent exercise and heavy lifting must, of course, be avoided. If you take things fairly easy and keep reasonably warm, the odds are that your muscle strain will be better within a matter of a few days or so.

Ligament and tendon strain

In Chapter 1 we explained that the ligaments are tough bands of connective tissue while the tendons ('sinews') are strong cords made of similar tough material.

Once again, these ligaments and tendons are subjected to colossal stresses when the joints of the backbone are forced beyond their normal range. When they are put 'on the stretch', the nerve endings within them start sending out 'pain signals' that immediately cause the muscles guarding the spine to tighten up and to stop the abnormal movement. That's why, when you try to force your spine beyond the point that causes pain, you find that you can't.

However, sometimes the body is caught unawares by a sudden movement. Before the protective muscles can stop things from going too far, the spine has been subjected to a stress that tears a ligament or tendon.

These tears are among the commonest causes of back pain. They tend to be provoked by sudden movements, and usually produce pain at the moment of the injury. Sometimes, however, pain does not arise until a few days later.

On the whole, doctors tend to treat ligament and tendon tears simply by advising the patient to rest as much as possible until the tear has healed.

Degenerative Joint Disease (Osteoarthritis) All of us get some form of ageing in our joints as we get older, and the joints between the spinal bones are no exception. Degenerative joint disease (DJD) affects about half the population by the age of sixty and probably nearly all people by the age of seventy. In other words, it's something that we all get eventually.

DJD isn't a serious thing, as a general rule, so it's unfortunate that it's known by the name osteoarthritis – a word that tends to terrify people because they think it means that they'll be crippled.

In fact, arthritis simply means inflammation of a joint – nothing worse than that. The common type of arthritis, associated with ageing, is nothing to do with the more severe forms of arthritis, and is most unlikely to cripple anybody.

59

Anyway, DJD, as we'll call it from now on, affects mainly the cervical and lumbar spine – that is, the neck and small of the back: the regions where most movement takes place. Many people over fifty get some degree of pain in these regions, and, particularly in the neck, they may notice some stiffness, or even 'grating' as well. From the neck, the pain may spread down the arms or sometimes up over the skull, while if the pain starts down in the lumbar region, it may spread down the backs of the legs.

DJD isn't a serious thing as a rule: the pain associated with it tends to come and go, and though an attack may be painful and annoying, it's usually soon over. Bed rest isn't necessary, and gentle activity may be helpful. Patients are sometimes encouraged to wear a collar if the trouble in the cervical spine is severe, and other lines of treatment include heat and the prescribing of anti-inflammatory drugs.

Disc trouble There's no doubt that disc problems do cause a lot of pain and suffering for some people, and when a disc does give trouble it can be quite difficult to treat.

We've explained in Chapter 1 that discs are the little shock absorbers between the bones of the spine. They don't slip – but what they sometimes do is to bulge outwards and press on a nerve root. This phenomenon is often referred to as a disc protrusion, or disc prolapse.

Lumbar disc trouble When most people talk about disc trouble they usually mean the discs in the small of the back – the lumbar region. Characteristically, what happens when somebody gets a disc prolapse here is that he bends forward suddenly, perhaps to pick up something from the floor, and then experiences a very severe pain low down in the back. Indeed, it may be so severe that he's unable to straighten up.

Either at that time, or a few days later, the pain often spreads down the leg, usually the back of the leg. It may be made worse by coughing or sneezing. Sometimes, however, the pain of a prolapsed disc is much less sudden and may come on gradually over a period of a few days.

Cervical disc trouble It is not widely realized that discs may also prolapse in the neck. Where this happens, the pain runs down into the arms instead of the legs.

The treatment of disc trouble is a very complicated business, and sometimes a rather frustrating one. Some, though not all, doctors believe that the 'core' of the disc has a natural tendency to return to its normal place, thereby relieving the pressure on the affected nerves. There are various ways of attempting to help this to happen:

Bed rest It's usual to recommend *absolute bed rest* in cases of sudden disc prolapse. The patient is usually advised by the doctor to stay flat on his back for at least a week, using a *very* firm mattress. Few mattresses are really hard enough, so it may be necessary to put a board underneath or to lie on the floor. *Rest is always the most important part of treatment.*

Plaster jackets and corsets These are no longer as widely used as they were, but neck supports (collars) are generally thought to be of more value than lumbar ones, and are still very frequently prescribed. They are believed to work simply by providing support and limiting movement. Though lumbar corsets are not so widely prescribed as they once were, it's interesting that a recent trial reported in the *British Medical Journal* seemed to indicate that they may give as good results as anything else.

Traction Stretching the spine was originally introduced with the idea that it would pull the spinal bones apart and so help the 'core' or the disc to slip back in. Nowadays, doctors disagree about this and many believe that its effect is to reduce muscle spasm and so improve spinal mobility.

Manipulation Originally the object of this procedure was to induce the disc 'core' to go back in, but many doctors would deny that it really does this! The subject of manipulation and osteopathy is discussed further in the next chapter.

Operation This is only very rarely necessary and usually when all other measures have failed. However, this doesn't mean that surgery is only advised when a patient is in danger of being crippled! It's important to stress, too, that such operations are very safe procedures these days and that they often lead to a complete return to normal activities.

Osteoporosis This is a 'thinning' of the bones which affects older people and especially women. After many years, the bones of the spine become so 'thinned' that they may collapse. The result is pain, loss of height and a 'bending forward' of the spine – which produces the condition known in women as 'dowager's hump'.

Treatment often involves giving high doses of calcium, or administering hormones. Fluoride therapy is sometimes used. A new and still controversial idea is that women should be given female hormone (oestrogen) replacement therapy continuously after the menopause in order to try to ward off this condition. Time alone will tell whether this works.

Ankylosing Spondylitis This is a disorder which is not all that uncommon in young men. It's also known as 'poker back' because of the fact that the low back pain it produces is associated with a progressive *stiffening* of the spine so that bending is difficult. The cause is unknown, but hereditary factors sometimes play a part. Other parts of the body may be involved as well as the spine. Physiotherapy and anti-inflammatory drugs help, and it's important to sleep on a hard, level bed.

Paget's Disease This is a disorder which quite often affects elderly people. The cause is still unknown, but the disease produces thickening, and sometimes pain, in various bones, including those of the back. No very effective treatment was available till quite recently, but new drugs are giving very promising results.

Non-diseases

Fibrositis Practically all non-medical people think there is a disease called fibrositis, but this isn't true. In years gone by, quite a lot of doctors did think that there was some slightly mysterious condition in which people's muscle *fibres* became inflamed ('-itis' means inflammation). It was thought that there were 'trigger spots' in the muscles of the back, and elsewhere, and that these inflamed spots were the source of the pain.

In practice, no one has ever been able to show, for instance with a microscope, that inflammatory changes in these so-called 'trigger-spots' really exist. Most people who were diagnosed as having fibrositis in the past probably either had a muscle or ligament tear, or else some degree of degenerative joint disease.

Rheumatism It may astonish you, but this isn't a disease either! It's a time-honoured word dating back several centuries, but today most doctors feel that it's pretty meaningless. The term 'rheumatic diseases' does provide a useful shorthand expression for all sorts of painful conditions of bone, joint, muscle and ligament, but there is no actual illness called rheumatism. But a lot of doctors still use the word when talking to their patients (but not to other doctors) simply because of the fact that it's a familiar and rather reassuring term. In these circumstances, the doctor uses it to cover a variety of conditions – muscle and ligament tears, degenerative joint disease and so on.

Lumbago Yet again, lumbago isn't a disease! It's an old term meaning simply pain in the lower part of the back (the lumbar region) from whatever cause. You'll frequently hear people say that they're 'suffering from lumbago' but this doesn't really mean anything, other than that they've got a pain in the lower back.

Sciatica And finally, sciatica isn't a disease either! In fact, it's a symptom – pain running down the back of the leg in the area which is served by the sciatic nerve. Like lumbago, it's a term used by doctors because their patients are familiar with it and recognize that it doesn't describe a serious condition. This nerve is a large 'communications channel' which runs down the back of the thigh; it is formed by the junction of a number of spinal nerves which leave the spinal cord, to pass between the bones of the back and join together deep in the buttock.

Pain felt down the back of the leg (sciatic pain) is very often due to something interfering with the roots of the nerves as they approach the spinal cord. Disc trouble can cause this, which is why a prolapsed lumbar disc is usually accompanied by pain running down the back of the thigh.

Other causes of sciatic pain include degenerative joint disease in the lumbar spine and irritation of the sciatic nerve or its roots. But let's repeat that sciatica isn't a disease in itself and if you've got this kind of pain, the next thing to do is to find out why.

Gynaecological backache For generations, any kind of backache in women was all too readily ascribed to disease of the female reproductive tract. But, in fact, in the words of one of this country's most distinguished gynaecologists, 'a woman with backache usually has something wrong with her back'. However, it's true that the womb and other pelvic organs are supplied by nerves which run up into the lower part of the spinal cord. This is why *period pain* and *labour pain* are so often associated with low backache. Most gynaecologists now think that it is very uncommon for any disease of the reproductive organs to produce backache, but pain felt over the lower spine may occasionally be due to a prolapse and can be associated with inflammatory disorders, such as cervicitis (inflammation of the neck of the womb), or salpingitis (inflammation of the tubes). Womb swellings, such as fibroids, may also sometimes produce backache. But if movement of the back is limited or painful, then it is most unlikely that the cause lies in the reproductive organs.

Psychological back trouble Like headache, back trouble can become worse as a result of emotional stress such as anxiety or bereavement. Pain is often more difficult to bear if you are worried about your job, have an upset in your personal relationships, or if you're under financial pressure.

And, of course, recurrent or chronic pain can itself be depressing, and the depression may make the pain feel worse, so that a vicious circle is created. If you *are* depressed or anxious, you may need additional help from your doctor in the way of a confidential chat about your problems, or perhaps some anti-anxiety or anti-depressant tablets.

6 The management of back pain

So far we've said a little about treatment, but we haven't explained how you *get* the treatment, and who gives it to you.

Well, let's stress at the start that *the first thing is to see your doctor*. He is the best person to decide what the line of treatment should be, and it's unwise to go off to masseurs or acupuncture specialists without seeing him first. As we said earlier, emergency calls are seldom necessary. Go to bed with aspirin and a properly padded hot water bottle, and phone him in the morning.

In fact, it's extremely difficult to predict just what sort of therapy will be best in any individual case of back pain – which is why it's really rather inadvisable to go off and select your own line of treatment without consulting your GP. So always take his advice before you do anything.

If your back is really bad, so bad that you find it difficult to walk, then don't go down to your doctor's surgery. Stay lying flat in bed on a firm mattress – if you haven't got one, get someone to push a board under the mattress, and telephone the doctor.

(Full advice on 'first aid' for the acute attack is given in Chapter 3.)

When you see your GP, he'll probably want to know the answers to several of these questions:

1 Have you had back trouble before?

2 When did the present pain start?
3 Did it come on suddenly?
4 If so, what were you doing at the time?
5 Had you put your back under any kind of stress in the few days before the pain came on?
6 Does your job or any spare-time activity involve any strain on the back?
7 Exactly where is the pain?
8 Does it run down your leg?

After that, he'll examine you. He'll look at your spine and will probably also want to do certain simple tests like lifting your leg off the examination couch or bed and seeing if this produces pain, and where.

From all this, he'll come to some conclusion about the cause of the pain, and will probably tell you what he thinks it is. Let's remind ourselves that it's most likely to be a simple muscle or ligament strain, with disc trouble coming a long way behind.

Now, what treatment will he suggest? Obviously, doctors differ in their approach to the various disorders that they're called on to treat, and nowhere is this more true than in the case of backache!

One particular problem for the doctor is that so far there have been few scientific trials of the various forms of therapy available for back pain, to discover how each kind of treatment compares with the rest. (One of the few major trials of this sort which have been published in recent years showed that in the management of low back pain, there is little to choose between four commonly used forms of therapy – manipulation, physiotherapy, pain-killing tablets, and the old-fashioned corset.)

Don't be surprised if what your doctor suggests is a little different from the advice we give here. Please be guided by him, because he knows you and therefore should have a reasonable idea of what's best for you.

There are several lines of treatment that he may suggest, to begin with:

Rest It's widely considered that rest is essential for *ligament strain*, so that the torn edges of the ripped tissues can heal together again.

In the case of *muscle strain*, rest and warmth are also a good idea. On the other hand, absolute immobility is definitely a bad idea. So patients are encouraged not to take to their beds but to keep mobile – though a few days off work may be necessary, and it's important to keep warm (see below).

In cases of suspected disc trouble, absolute bed rest is essential. If there is any doubt in the doctor's mind about whether a disc protrusion could have occurred, he'll almost certainly suggest that you stay in bed – on the aforementioned firm surface, of course, for at least a week.

In other conditions, e.g. Degenerative Joint Disease, rest is often advisable, but it rarely needs to be absolute, i.e. staying in your bed during the day. In fact, too much rest can be a bad thing, so follow your doctor's advice on this point.

Warmth Keeping warm is generally considered to be a good idea whatever the cause of your backache. Most kinds of pain feel worse in the cold. So if it's wintertime, and if your job is out in the open air or on cold premises, your GP may well have an extra reason for advising you to stay off work for a few days at least.

Heat Locally applied heat is good for many kinds of pain, and your doctor may advise this too. It isn't usually necessary to buy an expensive heat-lamp – a hot-water bottle wrapped in a towel and applied to the painful area of the back is usually adequate. In the case of anyone elderly, or slightly dopey from the effects of a sedative, a hot-water bottle must be used only with caution – remember that it can burn! Heat is also used by physiotherapists (see below).

Drugs It's very probable that your GP will give you a prescription for tablets or capsules, or for a bottle of medicine. The prescription is usually for an anti-inflammatory drug, which not only helps to damp down the 'angry' tissues round the site of the trouble, but also relieves pain to some extent. The most commonly prescribed anti-inflammatory drug of all is plain aspirin, which is still as useful as most of the complex drugs which have been developed by drug companies in recent years.

But don't take aspirin if it gives you tummy pain, or if you've had an ulcer. Prolonged self-treatment with aspirin is not a good idea, mainly because it may cause stomach irritation or internal bleeding.

Apart from anti-inflammatory drugs, many doctors prescribe *pain-killers*, and some try muscle-relaxants and enzyme preparations to relieve discomfort or aid healing: *sleeping pills and tranquillizers* are often used as well.

Massage Gentle rubbing is also good for most cases of back pain. By this we don't mean vigorous massage of the sort dished out by football team trainers, but just soothing rubbing with the fingertips over the painful area. Your wife/husband is the ideal person to do this for you, and your GP may give you a prescription for a 'warming' ointment or liniment to rub in, though in fact, the rubbing almost certainly does far more good than anything in the ointment! It's virtually impossible for the chemicals contained in many of these preparations to penetrate the skin to any significant depth.

The great majority of cases of backache will get better with treatment along the above lines, because they seem to be caused simply by muscle or ligament strains.

If things *don't* improve, however, your doctor will decide that it's time to seek further help. What sort of thing is he likely to suggest?

X-rays Sending you to the radiography department of the local hospital for an X-ray of your back may be helpful, especially if the pain has gone on for some time. X-rays in the *early* stages of back pain are not often of much use, so there's no point in trying to press your GP to order one!

The hospital specialist If the pain persists (or if it's very bad) your GP may send you to see a specialist at the hospital. He will probably be an *orthopaedic surgeon*, i.e. a doctor who does operations on bones and joints or *a specialist in physical medicine or rheumatology* (or perhaps a *neurologist*). This last group of doctors don't do operations, but in any case let's make it quite clear that only a minute proportion of all the people with backache ever come under the surgeon's knife. So just because you're going to hospital, it doesn't necessarily mean that there's any question of an operation!

The specialist, or indeed your GP, may suggest one of the lines of treatment that follows:

Physiotherapy is usually given in the physiotherapy department of your local hospital, though some physiotherapists do practise from their homes or consulting rooms, usually under the general direction of a doctor – the hospital specialist or your GP. Hospital physiotherapy is free under the NHS; private physiotherapists usually make quite modest charges.

Physiotherapy for people with back trouble may involve all sorts of techniques. Heat treatment is often used, and the reverse – application of ice – is also sometimes employed.

In many cases the physiotherapist also teaches gentle exercises to strengthen the back muscles and improve posture.

Hydrotherapy (immersion in warm water) is used in physiotherapy units fortunate enough to have a pool, and is also available at this country's relatively few spas and hydrotherapy hospitals. It is thought to be the temperature and the buoyancy support provided by the water that matters, and not the mineral content or so-called radioactivity. Back pain sufferers often get some relief of pain by going for a gentle swim at the local pool.

Traction, or stretching of the spine, is less commonly used than it once was, though some patients are still admitted to hospitals and kept 'on traction' for a period of time. This does at least ensure that they get plenty of rest. Other patients are given a period of spine traction each day as out-patients.

Massage is also used in physiotherapy departments, and most physiotherapists are now being trained in manipulation, which is dealt with below.

Manipulation Manipulation of the spine can be very helpful in some cases of backache (although it's certainly not necessary for most people). However, there are two important points to bear in mind:

First, there are a few situations where manipulation could make things worse, so it should only be used where serious disease has already been ruled out by a doctor.

Second, manipulation should only be carried out by someone who knows what he's doing – NOT your wife or one of your friends!

All right, well who *can* do manipulation?

A very few GPs have been specially trained in it, and also a relatively small number of *physiotherapists*. An increasing number of *hospital specialist doctors* (experts in orthopaedics, physical medicine and rheumatology) are using it. And also, of course, there are the osteopaths and chiropractors.

Who are osteopaths and chiropractors? Well, they are not doctors (as people sometimes think) but people who practise joint manipulation in order to try and relieve pain. Both types of therapy were started in the second half of the 19th century in America, and both remain a lot more popular in the USA than in the UK. Indeed, there are less than a hundred practising chiropractors who are members of the British Chiropractors Association, and only about three hundred osteopaths on the register maintained by the Osteopathic General Council. The basic difference between the two systems is that osteopathy tends to use an indirect method of manipulation, while chiropractic uses a direct one.

There are, however, about three thousand people who describe themselves as osteopaths in the UK, as *anybody* can call himself an osteopath, even if he hasn't had any training! The Osteopathic General Council, 16 Buckingham Gate, London, sw1 (Tel. 01–828 0601) will tell you whether any osteopath you are thinking of consulting is one of the three hundred on the Register: but, in practice, registered osteopaths can be identified by the letters mro after their names. In addition, a small number of doctors have taken osteopathic training, and these have the letters llco or flco after their names. The British Chiropractors Association, The Gate House, 1 Abbotswood, Guildford, Surrey, gu1 1vr, also maintain a list of their own members in the UK.

Vast numbers of people with back pain consult osteopaths or chiropractors, registered or unregistered, each year, and there is not the least doubt that many of them derive a lot of benefit from their manipulations. Anyone who has experienced immediate relief of pain after a successful osteopathic manipulation will not dispute this! But manipulation is not a magic remedy, so don't expect it to cure every case of backache. And it definitely shouldn't be used for 'general' illnesses.

Because osteopathy and chiropractic have never quite succeeded in achieving recognition in this country, they're not available on the Health Service. But registered osteopaths' charges are not excessive, and you can enquire in advance what the cost will be when you phone for an appointment. (Remember: most good osteopaths have long waiting-lists.)

Relationships between doctors and osteopaths or chiropractors have been very difficult in the past, and until quite recently a doctor who worked with such a practitioner would have been fairly certain to find himself up before the General Medical Council, the doctors' disciplinary body. But things are a good deal easier these days, and quite a lot of doctors, though not all, agree that there are benefits to be obtained from osteopathic or chiropractic treatment.

When you get back pain, however, it is best to *see your family doctor first*. If you want to consult an osteopath or chiropractor, do mention this to your doctor, rather than leaving him in the dark! In fact, many GPs won't have the least objection to your seeing an osteopath or chiropractor.

Injections Some doctors treat various types of back pain with injections around the site of the pain. Sometimes they inject a local anaesthetic, sometimes anti-inflammatory drugs called 'steroids'. Some doctors have found that injecting a steroid around the nerve root can relieve the pain. These 'epidural' injections, as they are called, require special skills and are only carried out in hospitals.

Supports Plaster jackets and corsets are still used in some cases of lower back pain (indeed, the trial we mentioned at the start of the chapter suggested that this 'old-fashioned' method may be as good as anything) while collars of various sorts are frequently prescribed for people with pain in the neck region.

Many people don't like wearing these supports, but if the doctor prescribes one for you, do please try to bear with it. By reducing the strain on the back, it may be of considerable help in relieving your pain and helping your body to heal. (Incidentally, don't fly to buy yourself a support corset – it should be prescribed by the specialist at the hospital.)

Well, that summarizes the treatment of back pain. But do remember that prevention is better than cure. When you get better from an attack of back pain, try to think about the factors that brought it on – the sort of factors we discussed in Chapter 2, like being overweight, or subjecting your back to unnecessary stresses during lifting or stretching or sitting. With a little bit of shrewd planning, you may be able to avoid ever having to go through the misery of backache again!

7 Learning to live with back pain

If you're a 'long-term' backache sufferer, how do you learn to live with it?

Well, it's not easy – let's admit that at the start. A lot of modifications have to be made to your life; it's simply no use just going on as before and hoping that everything will be all right, because it probably won't. Unless you re-think your life completely, you're going to be troubled very, very frequently by recurring episodes of back pain. Only by *planning* so as to avoid strain on your back can you reasonably hope to keep such episodes to a minimum.

Planning at work

Even if you've got really bad back trouble, it's most unlikely that you're going to have to give up work altogether. But *whatever* sort of job you do, you're going to have to make some modifications to the way you do it. When they're told this, some people just say flatly, 'I can't' – but that's a defeatist attitude. And if you go on thinking like that, then you're laying up trouble for yourself. It often takes several bad bouts of back pain before a person realizes that he *does* have to take a long look at his job and see how it can be altered so as to make it less stressful for his back.

Think particularly about any weights you have to lift – even such objects as typewriters and heavy ledgers can put a massive strain on the spine. Could somebody else move these loads for you? Or could these objects be positioned differently, so that they don't have to be moved around so much? Or could they perhaps be *slid* from place to place instead of lifted? And if all else fails and you *do* have to lift them, can you use a completely different lifting technique? (Safe methods of lifting are discussed in Chapter 4.)

If you're sitting in a chair for much of your time at work, think very hard about that. Is it really comfortable? Does it give firm support to your back? Does it seem the right height for you? If the answer to any of these questions is 'No', then it may be time for a change of chair!

If your employers are sensible people, they'll help you re-plan your job so that there's less strain on your back. (Better a re-planned job than somebody who's off work altogether.) Your Trade Union too may be helpful to you in this respect, and if your firm has a medical officer you should certainly have a chat with him about ways of lessening the strain on your back.

One useful trick, if you have a sedentary job, is to try to get up and move around every hour or so – remember, the human back just wasn't made for sitting at a desk for many hours at a time without a break!

Though this is not common, it does sometimes happen that a back pain sufferer simply *has* to change jobs altogether because of recurrent back strain. On the whole, it's probably better to do this sooner rather than later – before too much damage has been done to your back, and while you're still young enough to learn new skills.

Planning at home

The housewife with recurrent back pain has got to re-plan her life quite a bit, too. Admittedly the housework isn't just going to go away! But your husband and family can help you with it rather more than they used to, and often neighbours will be willing to lend a hand as well. When you're going through a bad bout of pain, your local Social Services department may be able to arrange a home help for you.

Perhaps most important of all for the housewife with a bad back is to *be realistic about housework*. Cleaning and polishing are not as vital as many people think, and it is far, far better to let the dust lie around for a few days than to put your back out by trying to get rid of the last speck! Taking it a bit easy on the cleaning isn't laziness – it's just common sense.

Remember, too, to make a point of sitting down (or lying down) and having a bit of a rest between difficult household tasks. Set yourself a target of, say, three or four such brief rests in a morning. Also very important is to get yourself a trolley. You know the kind of thing – they have them in supermarkets, but you can buy them through ironmongers. I'm always surprised that more people don't have these convenient trolleys in their homes to help them move heavy parcels, bring in the shopping and so on.

Finally, *stop lifting up the children*. Of course, this is impossible advice to follow if your kiddies are very tiny – but youngsters of three, four, five and upwards *don't* have to be picked up any more. Naturally, you have to explain to them that the fact that Mum (or Dad for that matter) doesn't give them piggy-backs isn't a sign that she doesn't love them: most children are very understanding once they realize that leaping up into an adult's arms can actually cause pain.

Getting help

The long-term back sufferer really does need help – not only from family and friends but often from outside organizations as well. Your doctor and your local Social Services department are the best people to advise you about what sort of help you need, and what facilities are available locally. Organizations which may be of particular assistance include the meals-on-wheels service (for people who are completely immobilized, even if only temporarily), the mobile library service, the local authority home help department, the Women's Royal Voluntary Service, and also the Red Cross.

The Red Cross are often very helpful, too, in telling you about *mechanical aids* which can make life easier for you. And frequently they, or the local Social Services department, have a small stock of such aids which they may be willing to lend you. In fact, with common sense, it often happens that a member of the family who's good at 'do-it-yourself' can improvise simple aids – for instance, a shoe-horn on the end of a pole, so that you don't have to bend over to get your shoes on; a stick with a hook, a net or a spike on it, so that you can get things without stretching; a pole lashed to a trowel so that you can do some gardening; or (best of all) one of those extending pincers (like a bit of trellis fencing), so that you can reach out and grasp things.

As far as gardening's concerned, a useful trick for the really severely disabled person (who hasn't been able to bend over for years) is to get somebody to build you *an elevated flower bed* – that is, one which is three feet above ground level. This takes a lot of doing, but can bring much pleasure to those who love growing flowers.

Keeping your spirits up

Above all, don't give up hope. Even if you've had really bad back pain for years and years, there is always a chance that it will improve or even go away altogether. Try not to get too depressed (though backache *can* be exceedingly depressing) because, as we learn more and more about the subject, the outlook for the sufferer from back pain is definitely improving all the time. In the next chapter, we'll talk about what's being done on the research front.

8 What about the future?

The really surprising thing about back pain is that *we know so little about it*. Basically, that's the reason why it is often so difficult to treat.

Why do we still know so little? Mainly because the interior of the back is so hard to study – it's not a hollow part of the body like the stomach, into which doctors can push telescopes or insert radio-transmitter capsules. Many's the time that your doctor would dearly love to open up your back to have a look at what's going on, and see just which tissues are strained or which structures are displaced.

But unfortunately he can't do that, except by asking you to undergo a surgical operation – which would only be justifiable in a few very severe and prolonged cases of back pain. And as we've explained earlier in this book, X-rays aren't usually all that much help to your doctor, either, because they only show the bones of the back, and not the softer tissues in which pain so often originates.

What is being done?

So, back pain research is far, far behind research into, say, heart or brain disease. But things are at last beginning to change, and in the past few years there has been much more interest in probing the secrets of the human back, and in meeting the challenge of back pain.

As far as pain relief is concerned, many new anti-inflammatory and pain-relieving drugs have been introduced, some of them with appreciably less side-effects than their predecessors. In one particular field (that of Paget's Disease) a new drug called calcitonin has been found which offers great promise in combating the disease process. So far there aren't many other drugs available for treating specific diseases, but at the time of writing a new preparation intended to benefit people suffering from osteoporosis is undergoing trials at Newcastle University.

What about the *investigation* of back pain? At Bristol, a team of doctors is using a new 3D X-ray machine which gives far better pictures of the bones of the spine than is possible with ordinary X-rays. (Incidentally, the machine which the Bristol team is using has been funded by the Back Pain Association.)

And at the University of Surrey, another research group is working on a project involving miniature radio transmitters which can give doctors information about stresses going on inside the body. We've said that these transmitters *can't* at present be inserted directly into the back – but the Surrey team are doing the next best thing: they're going to get volunteers to swallow the little 'radio pills' and they'll 'listen in' to them as they pass through the stomach and intestines. It's believed that the variations in internal pressure which the pills detect are directly related to the stresses which the spinal column is undergoing.

In the field of *manipulation*, there are now one or two research projects financed by the Department of Health. But perhaps the most encouraging trend of the last year or so has been the remarkable way in which doctors have become interested in this subject – which was previously considered 'unorthodox' or even downright suspect. Relations between doctors and registered osteopaths have improved, which is all to the good since both professions have much to learn from each other as far as back pain is concerned.

But, overall, there is no doubt that nothing like enough money is being spent on improving the outlook for backache sufferers. Perhaps this is because until recently back pain was almost considered a bit of a joke – except by those who had it! Money was available for all sorts of esoteric research projects, but *not* for finding out about this group of illnesses. This seems quite crazy when we know that back pain is among the most disabling and distressing of symptoms – and that it costs the country such a vast sum every year.

Still, there are signs that things are improving. Research workers in other parts of the world are investigating back pain problems. In this country, even as this book was being written, the Health Services Minister publicly admitted that the whole area of back pain was sadly under-researched. And following a campaign by the Back Pain Association, the Medical Research Council is understood to be looking at ways of boosting research programmes in this area. But the best and most encouraging recent development has been the Health Minister's decision to set up a working group of experts from several different specialities to advise on how best to diagnose, treat and above all *prevent* back pain.

What else can be done?

Apart from sheer 'medical' research, what is badly needed is far more research into what's called the 'ergonomic' aspects of back pain. This means the design of chairs, car seats, beds and furniture generally, and the study of the way that people's movements and posture (at work and in the home) affect their backs. At Guy's Hospital a team of doctors is making continuous recordings of the electrical impulses from the spinal muscles during different movements at work and trying to relate these to the onset of back pain. Anyone who looks at this subject will be appalled at how little is known about these matters and at the absolute blind ignorance with which most chairs, car seats and so on are designed and produced.

Perhaps the answer is that we, the public, should keep complaining about seating which gives us back pain (whether at the office, on public transport or anywhere else) and about furniture designs which seem to be created more to cause backache than to prevent it.

But, in the long run, the back pain epidemic in Britain is only going to be defeated by a massive research programme – a programme which is going to cost a lot of money. But it will be money well spent – for let's remind ourselves that back disorders cost this country a shattering £300 million each and every year in medical care, sickness benefits and lost production.

9 How common is back pain?

No one really knows for certain, but it's thought that *one-and-a-half million people every year* go to a doctor because of back trouble. And there are probably quite a lot more chronic back sufferers who soldier on year after year without consulting a doctor.

In fact, the problem is so serious that on any given day there are about *fifty six thousand men and women absent from work in the UK because of back trouble* – a pretty staggering figure.

Looking at it another way, let's imagine Wembley Stadium filled to capacity with about a hundred thousand people watching a football match. It's fairly certain that as many as three thousand of them will need to go to the doctor with back trouble during the next twelve months. *And about a hundred of them will be off work tomorrow, suffering the agonies of back pain.*

What is the cost of back pain?

Perhaps the best answer is 'an awful lot of money!' With more fit people in Britain disabled by back trouble than by any other illness, time lost to industry and business thanks to back pain is more serious than time lost through strikes!

In fact, back troubles result in the loss of at least fifteen million working days per year in this country – as opposed to the seven million working days lost in industrial disputes in 1973.

Even this staggering figure takes no account of women who work at home. Some manage to continue with their housework despite their aches and pains, but others may be incapacitated for a few days, several weeks, or be dogged by chronic discomfort and pain.

And if you tot up all the working days lost through all kinds of sickness, you find that seven per cent of the total is due to back trouble! Where the work is heavier, the incidence of backache is obviously a good deal higher, and people in certain occupations – nursing and mining, for instance – are particularly liable to run into trouble.

Among nurses, who spend a lot of their time lifting heavy patients, backache is so common that it's usual to talk about 'nursing back' as an occupational condition. And among miners, a survey at one colliery showed that nearly one-fifth of all time lost from work was due to back trouble – not perhaps surprising when you think of all the bending and lifting of heavy loads that miners have to do.

Other people who are at special risk of backache because of the hard physical work they do include dockers, building site workers, navvies, coalmen, sailors, brewery workers, dustmen, furniture movers, farmers and farm workers. Backache is also common in postmen – even though the loads they carry are not all that heavy; the constant strain of a sackful of letters on the spine over a period of many years is often enough to produce painful spinal disorders.

Another very large group of backache sufferers is made up by people who work in various forms of transport – everyone from bus drivers to airline pilots, in fact. They are affected not only because of the physical stresses of manipulating a large piece of machinery, but also because they have to spend so long in their seats (which, as we've said before, are often appallingly badly designed).

For the same reason, literally tens of thousands of 'chairborne' office workers are exceedingly liable to backache – including the junior typist and the senior executive. Even doctors are prone to back disorders, because of the fact that they spend so long sitting at their desks!

So, even in so-called 'lighter' work, backache is very common – and very costly. A few years ago a light engineering firm employing one thousand people worked out that back troubles cost them as much as £10,000 a year – or £10 for every single member of staff. Calculations show that if you apply these figures to the whole of business and commerce, *British industry is losing at least £200 m a year through back pain*.

That's a vast sum – enough to pay for a good many new hospitals and schools. But in fact it's only the beginning.

For how can you count the additional cost to the nation of all the medical treatment needed by back pain sufferers? The answer is – you can't.

But if between one and two million people go to the doctor each year because of back pain, then the cost of these consultations alone must run into millions of pounds. And when we consider that many, if not most, of these patients will have drugs prescribed by the doctor, which can easily cost £6 or so for a four-week course, then we can see how the national bill begins to mount up. Add to this the cost of all the specialized investigations and treatment that many people with back pain receive, e.g. X-rays, physiotherapy, and so on, and you can see that backache must take up a tidy sum of the £5,000 m spent by the National Health Service.

What else? Well, we haven't even begun to count the money that people spend for themselves on backache remedies and pain-killers, nor the money that they spend on private treatment from osteopaths, chiropractors, physiotherapists and doctors working outside the NHS.

But also very important is the cost that backache exacts in the home. In particular, we have to remember that it's not just the man or woman on the shop floor or in the office who gets back trouble: *it is the busy housewife, too.* Heaven knows what the cost is of having many, many thousands of housewives out of action every day because of back trouble!

So, we come back to our original question: how much does back pain cost the country? And our answer can still only be 'a very great deal of money!'

It was because of this and, of course, because of the widespread unhappiness and suffering caused by back troubles, that the Back Pain Association was set up as a charity to help promote and finance research into the causes, treatment and prevention of back pain disorders.

How much could back pain cost you?

Although back disorders are not likely to kill or permanently disable you, occasionally a person can lose his or her livelihood or have to change jobs because of recurrent back trouble.

But for the great majority of us, backache isn't likely to mean having to give up our jobs. What it can mean is a *temporary but significant loss of income.* Many, though far from all, people with back pain are advised by their doctors to stop work and go to bed for periods varying from a week to four weeks. Even after they're allowed to get up, they may perhaps be advised not to return to work for a further period of time that, again, might range from a few days to several weeks.

Ten years ago one researcher estimated that the cost to the individual sufferer was £66 for each spell of illness. With the inflation that's taken place since then – you can do the sums for yourself! Quite apart from the pain and distress caused by back trouble, it could put you off work for a week, two weeks, three weeks or more at some time in the future – *and the future could be tomorrow.*

Happily, there are ways of preventing back troubles. Let's say it again – *most back pain need never occur if people take sensible precautions against it.*

10 Summing things up

Back trouble and you

Almost certainly, you or one of your family will run into some kind of back pain one day.

At work, four out of five of the people you know will have back trouble at some stage.

But back pain isn't usually a symptom of some serious disease.

The back

The back seems to be a complicated structure but if you're a backache sufferer, it's worth getting to understand it.

It contains the body's main nerve communications channel (the spinal cord), which runs down through the many small bones that make up the spine.

These bones are surrounded by many muscles and ligaments which can easily tear.

Such tears are thought to be the commonest cause of back pain.

When things go wrong

Factors that can cause back trouble include:

Being overweight
Lifting heavy weights or lifting with a poor technique
Sitting badly, especially in a poorly designed seat

Driving, especially in an awkward posture and in a badly designed seat
Bending and stretching, at work or in the home
Poor posture generally
Sleeping in a bed that doesn't support your spine
Lack of adequate exercise

How to cope with an acute attack

Things you can do include:

Stopping whatever you're doing
Taking a mild pain-killer, such as aspirin or paracetamol
Going to bed – if in doubt, always do this
Keeping warm and cosseting yourself
Seeking skilled help after about twelve hours or so
Following the doctor's advice as to continuing care
Exercising your legs during the period you're confined to bed (to prevent clots in the leg veins)

How to prevent back pain

So, to prevent trouble arising in the first place, take the following commonsense precautions:

Don't get overweight.
Avoid heavy lifting.
If you must lift, use an approved technique.
Sit correctly, not round-shouldered and slouching.
Choose a chair that gives firm support to your spine.
When sitting at work surfaces, make sure the height of your chair is right in relation to the working surface.
If possible, avoid spending long hours behind the wheel of a car or lorry.
If you can't avoid driving, make sure you've got a good car seat.
And sit properly on it: not hunched up and cramped.

Arrange your workplace or your kitchen so that you don't have to bend and stretch unnecessarily.
At all times, try to keep your back reasonably straight, and don't let your shoulders slump forward.
Buy yourself a really firm mattress, preferably a new one from a reputable firm.
Make sure you get a reasonable amount of exercise every day, but – don't leap into violent and unaccustomed exercise!

The common causes of back pain

Don't try and diagnose your own back trouble. But remember that the more commonly encountered causes are:

Muscle strains
Ligament strains
DJD – or ageing of the joints of the spine
Disc trouble – far less common than people think
Osteoporosis – in older women especially
The following are NOT diseases:
Fibrositis
Rheumatism
Lumbago
Sciatica

What kinds of treatment are there?

Always begin by going to your GP and letting him decide on the line of treatment. Measures he may recommend to begin with include:

Rest
Warmth
Locally applied heat
Pain relieving and anti-inflammatory drugs
Massage

Further measures that may be needed include:
X-ray investigation
Referral to a hospital specialist
Physiotherapy
Manipulation
Injections
Supports

But prevention is better than cure. So, above all, remember that intelligent planning could prevent you from getting back pain in the first place.

Learning to live with back pain

Coping with long-term, persistent backache isn't easy. But it *can* be done if you remember certain things:

Plan ahead at work.
Change your scheme of working so that you don't have to lift things.
Make sure your chair is comfortable and gives good support to the spine.
When you've been sitting for an hour or so, get up and move around.
If you *have* to change jobs, do so earlier rather than later, while you're young enough to re-train.
Plan ahead at home, too.
Remember that the housework *isn't* as important as your back.
Get yourself a trolley for moving things.
Lift the children as little as possible.
Get help from local organizations.
See if there are any mechanical devices which can make life easier for you.
Keep your spirits up!

What about the future?

We know remarkably little about the causes and cure of back pain. But things are improving because:

New drugs are being developed.
Research is slowly getting under way.
There's much more interest in manipulation.
The Government admits that nowhere near enough money has been spent on the problem of back pain, and has asked a group of experts to advise.
And the Back Pain Association is doing everything it can to advance research on all fronts.

The cost of back pain

Back pain costs the country fifteen million working days a year.
It costs industry £200 m a year.
It could cost you several days', or even several weeks', pay.
It could put your wife out of action, unable to cook or look after the family for days or weeks.

Back Pain Association

The Back Pain Association is the only registered medical charity in the country whose sole aim is the promotion of research into the causes, cures and prevention of back pain. The Association has already embarked on an exciting research programme designed to answer the most urgent questions about the problems of back pain.

Through its industrial advisory service, the BPA is offering an important pioneer service to help industry and commerce to reduce the pain and disability caused by poorly designed machinery and working conditions.

The Association distributes information about modern methods of diagnosis and treatment and about new research, to those with a medical or professional interest in back pain, and is actively concerned to increase public understanding of how the problem can be avoided.

The Back Pain Association needs more money and more subscribers to help finance a worthwhile programme of research and education. Please help us with your donation, covenant, legacy or subscription.

How you can help to defeat back pain

I would like to make a regular donation
by covenant or banker's order

I enclose my donation of £

I would like to become a subscriber to the
BPA and receive copies of the Association's
newsletter, *Talkback*. I enclose my £5.00
for the subscription

I would like more information about the
Back Pain Association

Name ....

Address ....

....

....

Back Pain Association, Grundy House,
Teddington, Middlesex TW11 8TD
Telephone 01–977 1171

Arthur A. Michele
You Don't Have to Ache 40p

Chronic backache, hip pains, leg cramps : these are often caused
by muscular imbalance, which places unnecessary strain on the
body. Dr Michele, one of America's top orthopaedic surgeons,
shows how simple exercises can help you to restore your muscular
balance and so remove your pain.

Peter Blythe
Stress – The Modern Sickness 60p

Why is stress an ever-increasing problem ? How does the mind
convert stress into physical illness ? When can stress lead to a
broken marriage ? Is being over-weight a stress symptom ? These
and many other vital questions are discussed by Peter Blythe, a
practising psychotherapist and consultant hypnotist who examines
every aspect of normal living and shows where the build up of
anxiety-stress-tension plays a determining part in a variety of
illnesses

Malcom Jayson and Allan Dixon
Rheumatism and Arthritis 80p

Sooner or later we all suffer from some form of rheumatism This
excellent and highly informative book covers every aspect of
rheumatic and arthritic conditions, it is very readable, technically
explanatory and completely understandable to the layman, and the
detailed descriptions of specific diseases dispels the medical
mystique that many find frightening.

You can buy these and other Pan books from booksellers and
newsagents ; or direct from the following address :
Pan Books, Sales Office, Cavaye Place, London SW10 9PG
Send purchase price plus 20p for the first book and 10p for
each additional book, to allow for postage and packing
Prices quoted are applicable in UK

While every effort is made to keep prices low, it is sometimes
necessary to increase prices at short notice. Pan Books reserve the
right to show on covers new retail prices which may differ
from those advertised in the text or elsewhere